AMAZING STRENGTH OF VEGETABLES AND FRUITS

TAYLOR FRANCIS

Disclaimer

Table of Contents

INTRODUCTION

Concerning fruits and veggies

Vegetables and fruits have to be a major component of your everyday diet. They are nutritious by nature and include vitamins and minerals that may support your well-being. They may also aid in the prevention of certain illnesses.

Eating more fruits and vegetables as part of a healthy, well-balanced diet and an active lifestyle will benefit the majority of Australians. Fruits and vegetables come in a wide range of kinds, and there are several methods for preparing, cooking, and serving them.

Amazing strength of vegetables and fruits.

When fruits and vegetables are in season, they are best purchased. If not, consider

using canned or frozen veggies, which are equally nutrient-dense and cost-effective.

A minimum of five servings of vegetables and two servings of fruit should be consumed daily. Make a variety of color choices.

Start off cautiously with fruits and veggies you like eating if you're not one of those people. Try varied approaches to preparing, serving, and flavoring them. Additionally, you may hide them in curries, minced meats, and sauces.

CHAPTER ONE

WHY VITAMINS AND MINERALS ARE THE SOLUTION.

Many of us wish we had better abs, greater energy, and more concentration. Similarly, we often find ourselves wishing we had better hair or skin. We want more restful sleep at night and a somewhat easier time waking up (the latter two are connected, incidentally!).

As a result, several businesses have emerged, all centered on improving our performance, appearance, and sense of well-being. We shell out enormous sums of money for gym memberships, cosmetic products, and sleep aids. We experiment with a lot of strange stuff, including wearing blue-blocking sunglasses all day, sleeping on a bed of soft spikes (yeah, it works!), and wearing energy-healing crystals (which are about as effective as hoping very hard!).

We attempt these things out of desperation and a search for solutions. We are open to trying anything. And every time, we hold out hope that we're going to find the solution and realize our greatest potential.

We're hoping that ONE of these solutions will work and make us feel amazing because we know we can do this. However, very few of these tactics have any discernible impact.

The issue? We're making things too complicated. And a big part of this is because we are constantly inundated with marketing material. All it takes to feel and look better is knowing the fundamentals!

Think about the lifestyle and nutrition that you most likely lead at the moment. If you can relate to any of these things, raise your hand:

You consume an excessive amount of processed foods and prepared meals; you only visit the gym three times a week and are not very active the rest of the time; you don't get enough sleep; you are chronically stressed out from work, family, and financial obligations; you spend a lot of your free time watching cartoons on the couch; you spend more than eight hours a day staring at a bright computer screen with a hunched back; You breathe unhealthy smog-filled air;

you drink tainted tap water; and you hardly ever go outside.

Although this paints a fairly dismal image, it is accurate for MANY of us. We overindulge in sweet foods, sleep little, consume too few vegetables, and experience constant stress. Then, we question why we don't feel complete!

The fact is that our contemporary lives are just plain bad for our health, even if you answered the majority of these questions correctly.

This is accurate, all the way down to the fact that most of us lead too cushy lives and have "adapted" to a pleasant, domesticated way of life, so our bodies have forgotten how to handle hardship or stress.

Take a trip outside, for example. The majority of us just don't do this often enough, which means we aren't receiving the vital stimulation of sunshine, which aids in stimulating the body to make vitamin D, which in turn controls hormone synthesis, mood, sleep, and even hunger!

Our body loses part of its natural rhythm and various functions are disrupted in the absence of that crucial input, which is referred to as an "external zeitgeber" in the scientific literature.

There is, however, one very important advantage to being chilly. Being outside increases testosterone levels fortifies the immune system, and even enhances our capacity to control our body temperature, even in the absence of sunlight.

Given that we seldom exercise this aspect of our health, is it any surprise that we always feel "stuffy"?

Our bodies yearn for activities like going barefoot on the ground, which strengthens the tiny muscles in our feet, and diving into the water and holding our breath, which strengthens our lungs and balances our carbon dioxide levels. And that's not what we're providing them.

And as a consequence, our bodies are severely degrading. A wolf in the wild is comparable to an obese, pampered house dog. What is more healthful?

That domestic dog is YOU. In addition to a very demanding lifestyle and little sleep...

THE SOLUTION IS TO START WITH VEGETABLES AND FRUITS

The answer is to start with fruits and vegetables. How come?

All right, so it's all very well on my end that I advise you to work out all day, eat healthily, and swim for a long time in ice-cold water in the morning. The issue is that we don't have time for it, and our bodies aren't made for it these days.

It takes a lot of effort and may get fairly hard to even repair your diet, including getting rid of all that unnecessary processed food, cutting calories overall, increasing fiber, and lowering simple carbohydrates. For this reason, addressing one of the most pressing problems in contemporary life is the ideal place to start. I.e., insufficient micronutrients.

Amazing strength of vegetables and fruits.

Micronutrients are active components found in food such as vitamins, minerals, fatty acids, amino acids, and antioxidants that the body employs for a multitude of functions. Many individuals are unaware that our diets shape who we are. This is a common phrase, yet a lot of people mistake it for a metaphor. However, no—your body truly rebuilds your body using the nutrients it receives from your diet.

For instance, calcium and magnesium are partially used to make your bones. They also support the strength of your teeth, nails, and connective tissue, including tendons and ligaments. Collagen—which is included in bone broth—benefits connective tissues in a similar way to how it benefits skin.

Then, you would become the healthiest and most productive version of yourself if you could only include more fruits and vegetables in your diet. You could then have the motivation and strength to finish the remaining tasks as a result.

Vegetables and fruits may even speed up your metabolism, enabling you to burn off a lot more fat!

It's not hard to increase your diet of fruits and vegetables, as we'll see throughout the remainder of this book. If you are strategic, you can drastically improve your health and well-being by implementing a few easy adjustments.

Several additional remarkable and intricate ways that fruits may enhance your health and performance will also be covered in this

Amazing strength of vegetables and fruits.

book, some of which can completely change the way you feel and look.

You'll be fully aware of the fruits and veggies you need to treat any ailments you may be experiencing, as well as how to get them.

Let's get started.

CHAPTER TWO

An Introduction to Vitamins

Let's take a closer look at the particular advantages of fruits and veggies before moving on. Naturally, checking the vitamin content is the best place to start.

The fact that vitamins were discovered less than a century ago may surprise you. Doctors recognized that certain diets benefited specific physical ailments before they were formally identified, but they did not know why.

In 1975, for instance, the British Navy kept a stock of limes on hand because medical professionals discovered that consuming a certain quantity of lime juice or eating the fruit every day prevented sailors from developing scurvy.

But Casimir Funk, who first worked in the UK and subsequently in the USA, did not coin the name "vitamines," which eventually became vitamins, until 1912.

Since then, research on vitamins has advanced, and although most people are aware of the names of the most popular vitamins, we may not always be aware of their functions. Two categories of vitamins exist. These vitamins are water-soluble and fat-soluble.

The vitamins that the body can store are known as fat-soluble vitamins. This implies that vitamins may be kept in the body and used as needed, even if you do not utilize them all in your diet.

The apparent benefit of fat-soluble vitamins is that you are less likely to get a deficit if one of these vitamins is momentarily absent from your diet. These vitamins have the drawback that if you take too much of one of them, your body won't be able to get rid of the excess, which might lead to a vitamin overdose.

Vitamins Soluble in Fat

The four fat-soluble vitamins that are most well-recognized are vitamins A, D, E, and K.

Vitamin A maintains the mucous membranes' suppleness, smoothness, and moisture content in addition to helping to keep the skin moisturized. Along with supporting healthy bone development and reproductive system function, it also aids in maintaining normal vision in low light. Liver, eggs, butter, and whole milk are good sources of vitamin A. Carotenoids, a kind of vitamin A, are present in fruit and vegetables that are red, yellow, and dark green.

The body needs vitamin D to absorb calcium. As a result, it shares responsibility with calcium for the health of teeth and bones. Both, nevertheless, are interdependent and necessary. 'Fortified' foods like cereals and fat spreads often have vitamin D added to them. Since sunlight is the primary source of vitamin D, it is frequently referred to as the "sunshine vitamin."

The maintenance of a healthy neurological system, reproductive system, and muscles is attributed to vitamin E. Plus, it's an antioxidant. Because it dissolves in fat, the body stores it and uses it to shield cells from the destructive effects of free radicals, which may harm other cells in the body.

Nuts, wheat germ oil, whole grains, and green leafy vegetables are good sources of vitamin E. It is believed that taking too many vitamins might be harmful. The primary factor for blood clotting is vitamin K. You would risk dying from bleeding to death if you didn't have it every time you cut yourself.

Additionally, this vitamin forms bone and kidney tissues. Liver, cheese, cereals, dark green leafy vegetables, and fruit are good sources of vitamin K. Friendly microorganisms in the intestines also produce it.

Vitamins that are soluble in water cannot be kept in the body. It follows that if you take too much of any of these vitamins, the excess is eliminated via urine. One benefit of vitamins that are soluble in water is that overdosing is unlikely to occur.

Because these vitamins cannot be stored, you may need to take them in bigger doses. Your body does not keep a backup supply of any of these vitamins, so if your diet is lacking in any of them, even for a short period, you may experience the symptoms of a vitamin deficiency.

Vitamins Soluble in Water

The B vitamin family as a whole and vitamin C are the two most well-known water-soluble vitamins. Ascorbic acid is another name for vitamin C. It supports the integrity of the body's connective tissues, which include the bone structure, muscle, and fat.

In addition, it is an antioxidant, promotes the growth of new cells in wounds, and aids in the body's absorption of iron. Vitamin C also helps the body fight illness by strengthening the immune system.

Vegetables, fruit juices, and fruit are good sources of vitamin C. The vitamins in the B group include B1 (thiamin), B2 (riboflavin), B3 (niacin), B6 (pyridoxine), and B12 (cyanocobalamin). The main goal of this vitamin group is to maintain the body's optimal functioning.

The body needs vitamin B1 to properly metabolize lipids, alcohol, and carbs into energy. Nuts, seeds, lean pork, and unrefined grains are good sources of this vitamin.

B2 keeps hunger in check and aids in the body's use and digestion of proteins and carbs. Eggs, fish, poultry, pork, and milk are sources of vitamin B2. Both brewer's yeast and dark leafy greens are excellent providers of this nutrient.

B3 is necessary for healthy development and for allowing oxygen to enter bodily tissues. It is also in charge of maintaining a balanced appetite. Meat, cereals, and bread that have been fortified are sources of vitamin B3.

The B6 vitamin is in charge of helping our bodies absorb nutrients and energy from our diet. By lowering blood levels of excess homocysteine, it helps prevent heart disease. Soya beans, almonds, eggs, whole grains, salmon, lamb, wine, chicken, and milk are among the foods that are good sources of B6.

Red blood cell production in health is aided by B12. Additionally, it permits the body to communicate amongst nerve cells, allowing us to move, hear, think, and carry out our regular daily tasks. Bacteria in the small intestine of the body produce it.

This vitamin is added to a variety of meals, such as cereals, and even though it dissolves

Amazing strength of vegetables and fruits.

in water, the liver can retain it. Poultry, fish, milk, meat, and eggs are sources of B12.

Eating a balanced diet is the greatest method to make sure you get enough of the water- and fat-soluble vitamins. Seek counsel from a physician if you believe you could be lacking in any vitamins.

CHAPTER THREE

A GUIDE TO MINERALS AND OTHER AMAZING NUTRIENTS IN FRUITS AND VEGETABLES

While fruits are often rich in vitamins, veggies tend to be a better source of minerals; nonetheless, both fruits and vegetables are rich in both.

What distinguishes a vitamin from a mineral would thus be a good place to start.

In contrast, minerals are inorganic, whereas vitamins are organic and hence extremely volatile (they may be broken down by things like heat, oxygen, and acid). A mineral might indeed be a metal or a rock—things you would never truly consider to be essential components of who you are.

Minerals are, in fact, essential to the human body's proper operation. For instance, the body needs iron as a necessary mineral to produce hemoglobin, which is what gives red blood cells the ability to transport oxygen throughout the body.

Energy would not be able to be distributed throughout the body for the many vital processes that take place, such as breathing and digestion, without this mechanism.

In general, minerals have a significantly more important function in the tougher and more structural components of the human body. Minerals, for instance, make ligaments, tendons, and bones.

But minerals are involved in conduction as well. After all, the body is powered by electricity, and keeping our muscles and brains functioning properly depends on maintaining the proper charge.

Because of this, an imbalance between sodium and potassium may lead to cramping because the body cannot properly communicate with the muscles. Similar to this, low calcium levels might impair strength as they are required to manage the charge in the muscle cells.

Were you aware? Based on the seed or stone, you may differentiate between a fruit and a vegetable. They are absent from vegetables! Some unusual food classifications are as follows: cucumber, avocado, coconut, tomatoes, and so on.

Additional Crucial Micronutrients

Fruits and vegetables are a great source of the two other necessary elements in addition to vitamins and minerals. necessary amino acids and necessary fatty acids are the two essential nutrients.

The word "essential" refers to the fact that certain nutrients must come from our diets since the body is unable to produce them. Maybe this also indicates the extent of the issue, as 99 percent of us do not understand things that way!

What then are these nutrients doing?

As it happens, amino acids serve as the building components of proteins. Our bodies will then break down those component pieces to repair our tissue. We acquire a lot of them from meat. We are what we eat, as this book's introduction demonstrated!

For this reason, proteins and amino acids in general are crucial for bodybuilders and athletes who want to gain muscle mass.

According to research, athletes should consume one gram of protein for every pound of body weight. Other advantages of protein include its greater resistance to being converted to fat and its thermogenic action, which causes digestion to burn calories!

As a result, a lot of individuals will be working hard to obtain meat sources of protein and will consume a lot of chicken to gain muscle mass. This might become rather laborious! However, they overlook the fact that fruits and vegetables (albeit veggies are somewhat better in this regard) also contain protein.

Consider the amount of protein in the broccoli that is served with the chicken in addition to the amount you received from the protein shake and the chicken.

In addition to their many other functions in the body, amino acids are needed to make digestive enzymes, neurotransmitters (chemicals that are found in the brain), and many other things. They are also capable of generating.

Lastly, necessary fatty acids are present in fruits and vegetables. These are essential fats that aid in our increased absorption of other fruits and vegetables and provide a host of other practical advantages, including improving brain function (a significant portion of the brain is composed of fat!).

Amazing strength of vegetables and fruits.

One of the most potent necessary fatty acids available, omega 3 offers an enormous array of wonderful advantages. Although we often associate omega 3 with fish, it may also be found in significant quantities in seaweed, hemp seeds, walnuts, kidney beans, soybeans, and other foods.

CHAPTER FOUR

Nutrients and Fruits for Enhancing Athletic Performance

Chances are, when you consider a diet for muscle growth, you immediately think of the traditional choices. You'll probably concentrate mostly on protein-rich foods like eggs, tuna, and poultry. Steamed rice and meta should be the only foods an athlete eats, right?

However, many other foods are beneficial for increasing muscle mass and enhancing athletic performance. In reality, a balanced diet that includes a variety of food categories is crucial for bodybuilding, sprinting, swimming, long-distance running, and all other forms of athletic endeavors. You must eat your fruits and veggies.

Are you considering using supplements to improve your sports performance? You may be surprised to hear that eating more fruits and vegetables might be more cost-effective and beneficial to your health in several different ways!

These are a few instances.

The Best Fruits and Vegetables for Increasing Sports Performance

Beets-

Amazing strength of vegetables and fruits.

Without a doubt, beets are one of the most crucial veggies for athletes of all stripes who want to gain muscle.

This is because beets are among the foods that increase nitric oxide levels the best in the world. A naturally occurring "vasodilator" is nitric oxide. This implies that it may induce the arteries and veins in the blood to dilate, or expand, which will promote the body's natural flow of nutrients and oxygen.

As a consequence, during exercise, the muscles get more oxygen and energy as well as more nutrients to promote recuperation. This will enable you to run further, carry heavier weights for longer repetitions, and recover more quickly.

Crayons

Although they are often portrayed as the bad guys, carbohydrates are essential for both general physical exercise and muscular growth. Because potatoes are low in calories, rich in fiber, and high in vitamin C, which promotes recovery, they make an excellent option for carbohydrates. If you eat this after working out, the energy will go directly to your muscles instead of your waist.

Sprouts

In addition to having a high protein content, spinach is an excellent source of phytoecdysteroids. They are not the same as anabolic steroids, but they could have a comparable impact; in fact, some research suggests they are an effective way to promote testosterone production and muscle growth.

Lettuce

The vegetable with the most calcium is kale. Calcium is beneficial to your exercise routine since it not only helps to build stronger bones but also connective tissue and stronger contractions that provide you with more explosive power.

Because it's low in calories and rich in protein, kale is a popular vegetable right now. It's a pity it costs so much, however!

mushies

Amazing strength of vegetables and fruits.

Although they belong in the same aisle and are suitable for vegans, mushrooms are acceptable to include in this list even if they aren't fruits or vegetables. Mushrooms provide several other health benefits and advantages in addition to being a fantastic source of protein. They have a ton of minerals, help speed up the healing process after exercise, and much more!

It's only a matter of time before we see protein smoothies with mushrooms appearing in health shops!

The presence of vitamin D in mushrooms is yet another fantastic advantage. They are really among the few dietary sources of vitamin D! (Oily fish is another).

This is significant because, being one of the primary anabolic hormones for fat-burning and muscle growth, testosterone is produced with the help of vitamin D, which is regarded as a master hormone regulator. Furthermore, it has recently been shown that vitamin D has much greater immune-boosting and cold- and flu-preventive power than even vitamin C. Any athlete understands that having a cold may completely ruin their training schedule, which can be the difference between success and failure!

Carapace

In general, carrots are healthful and a fantastic source of vitamins A, C, and K. But what's truly intriguing about them is the lutein, which may help boost your energy levels and improve your mitochondria's function!

Your cells' energy factories, or mitochondria, are responsible for converting glucose into ATP, which is your body's useable type of energy. Glucose is a sugar that is derived from carbohydrates. This indicates that you can run faster and burn more calories even while you're at rest if you eat carrots and other foods high in lutein!

In one research, rats were given lutein (which requires a fat source, like milk), and it was seen that the rats started to run in their wheel for extended periods of their own will, burning much more fat in the process.

Fruits

Amazing strength of vegetables and fruits.

Vitamin C, which is abundant in apples, is also essential for strengthening the immune system and enabling athletes to work harder and longer without fail. When combined with zinc, vitamin C also promotes the healing of muscular tissue, raises serotonin to assist with mental recuperation, and even boosts the synthesis of nitric oxide and testosterone.

In addition to all of this, apples have a high fiber content, which may benefit blood pressure, bowel motions, food absorption, and other health issues. In addition, fiber is essential for maintaining a healthy microbiome, which supports several other benefits including improved mood, weight reduction, and a robust immune system.

CHAPTER FIVE

AMAZING SUPERFOOD VEGETABLES AND FRUITS FOR ENERGY, BEAUTY, MOOD, AND MORE

You don't care about losing weight, then? Maybe you're OK with your current size already? (Well done!)

Perhaps you're not that athletic? Perhaps you don't seem to have any health issues.

Look, everyone should eat fruits and veggies. And to further emphasize that point, consider these more instances of fruits and vegetables having a wide range of distinct health advantages.

Broccoli and Leafy Greens: Benefits for Beauty and Pregnancy

Indeed, eating fruits and veggies may improve your appearance. That holds for even something as basic as your common broccoli!

Compared to some of the other superfood fruits and vegetables on our list, broccoli may seem a bit less "exotic." Don't let that deceive you, however; this is still a highly nutrient-dense meal that everyone needs to consume more of.

First of all, broccoli has a high fiber content and may benefit your digestive system, bowel motions, and many other aspects of your health. Broccoli is also particularly rich in iron, calcium, collagen, fiber, potassium, vitamin C, and a host of other nutrients.

Let's get started by discussing collagen. We all need this, but not many of us get it. It has been shown that collagen helps prevent leaky gut syndrome, strengthens nails, lessens back discomfort, fights Alzheimer's disease, improves skin elasticity, and overall toughens up your tendons, ligaments, and bones.

This explains why foods like bone broth are so beneficial to humans. Furthermore, more recent studies point to a compelling explanation for why collagen may be so crucial. Scientists now believe that consuming animal bones would have been the primary source of sustenance for humans in the past. It is argued that hunter-gatherers may not have had the necessary tools to pursue enormous game. But we were highly skilled at finding and pursuing our prey.

The most plausible scenario would have been that humans would have often followed antelopes and other animals to the point where lions and tigers attacked and killed them. After that, they would have removed all of the flesh from those animals, leaving just the bones. At that point, the crafty and clever humans would have appeared, used our tactile hands to crack apart the bones, and consumed the nourishing collagen from inside.

If this is accurate, then our environment throughout evolution included consuming a lot of the components that make up bone. And we are suddenly thrown into a world where these vital nutrients are very uncommon. In that instance, broccoli could be much more advantageous than we first thought!

It is undoubtedly advisable for expectant moms to increase their intake of broccoli and other green vegetables. This is because broccoli and a variety of salad greens are excellent providers of folate, which is advised for all moms to consume.

Pregnancy difficulties may arise from inadequate folate intake, which is why many moms attempt to artificially boost their folate intake by using pregnancy supplements.

At this point, it's critical to highlight the substantial benefits of increasing your dietary intake of nutrients rather than using supplements. Although supplements might be beneficial, the word itself gives the game away. These are meant to be included in your daily diet.

In other words, rather than being used in place of your usual diet, they should be taken in addition to it. Since nutrients from your food are coupled with many other nutrients, lipids, fibers, and other components, they are significantly more effective than those taken as pills.

When combined, they enhance the essential components' absorption, increasing their effectiveness. It's important to understand that since the human body develops while consuming these meals, it is best suited to absorb the nutrients in this manner.

It is not intended to eat artificially supplied nutrients. For this reason, a lot of people advise against taking vitamin pills on an "empty stomach." They just function better as meals.

Testosterone, Weight Loss, and Other Benefits of Cayenne Pepper

In the meanwhile, cayenne pepper is an excellent weapon in the fight against inflammation. Due to its anti-inflammatory properties, this chemical, which gives food its fiery flavor, is often found in ointments and lotions. Because it depletes nerve cells of the chemical "substance P," it is also a frequent pain reliever. If you do have a problem like fibromyalgia or arthritis, substance P is an excellent addition to your diet since it promotes both inflammation and pain perception.

Flavonoids and carotenoids are also abundant in cayenne. These antioxidants work to stop cellular damage, which helps to fight inflammation even more.

Moreover, cayenne pepper offers many additional noteworthy advantages. For example, it is an excellent appetite suppressant, so if you have trouble sticking to a diet, you may find it a bit easier to maintain discipline and, perhaps, start to lose weight.

Moreover, cayenne pepper could aid in better digestion. This is important since improved digestion increases your energy and reduces pain while also improving your body's ability to absorb nutrients from meals. This implies that all of the advantages you are now reaping from the other superfoods on this list will intensify. Moreover, studies have shown that cayenne pepper raises testosterone. Naturally, this hormone—which the majority of us refer to as the "male hormone"—is in charge of the male sex drive and a host of other characteristics that set males apart from women. Men who have more testosterone have greater tone in their muscles, store less fat, become more aggressive, recover more quickly, strengthen their immune systems, and more.

Men who don't obtain enough testosterone will show symptoms of poor mood, low energy, reduced sex desire, and sadness. They also battle decreased muscle mass and weight growth. On the other hand, males with high testosterone display robust, toned bodies combined with the characteristics of the traditional "alpha male."

This explains why so many men attempt to increase their natural testosterone levels by using steroids and other pharmaceuticals, even though these substances come with several health risks and cautions.

The concerning aspect is that male testosterone levels are rising globally at a rate of 1% per year. This is caused by several issues (specific plastics and our generally sedentary lives), as well as the use of feminine products and their effect on our water supply. However, nutrition also has a significant impact. It's time to start consuming somewhat more cayenne pepper and less processed meals.

Elderberry as an Anti-Inflammatory

Nutrient-rich berries include elderberries. Again, this is a fruit that isn't often included in our diets, so you may want to try to include it again.

The majority of us eat the same handful of fruits and vegetables every day, that much is certain. Nonetheless, by doing so, we guarantee that we get a large amount of nutrients while excluding certain others. The most diverse diet—one that incorporates the most variety of fruits, vegetables, meats, herbs, and other foods—is the optimal diet. What benefits can elderberry provide you, then?

Amazing strength of vegetables and fruits.

Many ancient societies, like the Ancient Egyptians, have used elderberries as a supplement or medicinal since prehistoric times. We now know that these fruits are rich in flavonoids, particularly our buddies the anthocyanins, which are potent antioxidants similar to resveratrol.

Elderberries have also been shown to assist in increasing cytokine production. These are the messenger molecules that our bodies use for immune system regulation. While anti-inflammatory cytokines aid in reducing inflammation, pro-inflammatory cytokines contribute to its growth. All of this is crucial since it essentially guarantees that the body can appropriately control how it reacts to infections and illnesses as well as aid in the healing of wounds and injuries.

Amazing strength of vegetables and fruits.

Although many of us believe that inflammation is always negative, it promotes healing by bringing more nutrients to the damaged region and aids in the destruction of infections before they have a chance to spread. The issue arises when this reaction gets crazy.

It turns out that elderberry may be quite helpful in the fight against allergies for similar reasons!

Elderberries may also be used to treat infections, colds, and a variety of other ailments because of their exceptional efficacy in battling and eliminating microorganisms. The most intriguing thing of all is that the little berries have strong antiviral properties that have been shown to really "deactivate" viruses.

Amazing strength of vegetables and fruits.

These function by stopping the viruses' utilization of their haemagglutinin spikes to penetrate cell membranes, thereby rendering them almost inactive. As a result, they are very successful in both treating and avoiding conditions like rhinitis.

Naturally, berries also often contain the same amount of vitamins and minerals.

CHAPTER 6

ANTIOXIDANTS' IMPACT ON LONGEVITY

In addition to being present in many supplements, antioxidants are also naturally occurring in our food. These days, antioxidants are somewhat of a buzzword. A variety of Naka Herb supplements, as well as antioxidant vitamins and minerals, are quite well-liked.

What causes this to be the case? And just what are antioxidants exactly? We'll briefly examine how cells function, how they age, and the significance of antioxidants in this section.

Although there are many components to our cells, in this case, you just need to be aware of the cell wall and the nucleus. Naturally, the component of the cell that keeps everything together and gives the cell its spherical shape is the cell wall, which is encircled by mitochondria.

In the meanwhile, the nucleus—also known as the "control center"—is the hub of the cell. The 'blueprint' that instructs a cell on how to act, what to look like, and where other significant cells should go in the body is found in this area.

Unfortunately, our bodies also contain "free radicals," which is where the antioxidant vitamins, minerals, and supplements from Naka Herbs come in handy. Free radicals are essentially chemicals that circulate throughout the body and harm cells. They result from a variety of processes, including breathing (since oxygen is reactive and breaks down cells) and excessive sun exposure (UV rays from the sun are radioactive and may also break down cell walls).

Becaussmall little amounts of damage may ultimately accumulate to the point that it is apparent to the unaided eye, that free radicals inflict significant harm to the body, including aging of the skin's cells. This is why prolonged sun exposure will give you a nice tan in the short term, but in the long run, it will make your skin seem leathery and wrinkled.

More significantly, however, these free radicals will ultimately penetrate the cell walls completely, which will allow them to enter the nucleus, which contains the DNA. If they manage to get past this, they have the potential to harm your real genetic code, which might lead to mutations that alter cell expression and impair its ability to function. Because cells divide during mitosis, which is the process by which they reproduce, you will have two defective cells as a result of the cell dividing. While purchasing herbs online may support your immune system's efforts to fight this, it would be preferable if it could be avoided. Because those dead cells might ultimately cause whole organs to fail due to cancer that develops from them as they spread.

This may be accomplished with the aid of antioxidant vitamins and minerals found in fruits, vegetables, and even supplements. These nutrients work by scavenging free radicals before they have a chance to do any harm. Then, this will assist in preventing cancer and slow down your visible aging process. Not bad!

CHAPTER SEVEN

Using fruits and vegetables to successfully improve your health is covered.

By now, you need to be fully aware of the top motivations to make sure your diet is obtaining enough fruits and veggies. These micronutrients provide a multitude of health benefits, and if you are experiencing symptoms such as fatigue, mood swings, illness, or depression, you are probably lacking in one or more of them. And considering that the great majority of individuals these days DO have some kind of deficit, this shouldn't be shocking.

How should you be integrating these fruits and veggies gradually is the following issue. Do any negative aspects? Exactly how many do you need? Could you simply take a vitamin pill in its place?

The Question Is: How Much Fruit and Vegetable Do You Need?

You've likely heard that your daily intake should aim for at least five different fruits and vegetables. Numerous governments and health groups recommend this broad guidance. Some groups have raised this figure to seven. Although it is sound counsel, it is also subjective.

By that, what do I mean? That it has no foundation at all!

Amazing strength of vegetables and fruits.

Vegetables and fruits are not naturally healthful. Because they are fruits and veggies, they are not healthy for you. Instead, the reason they are healthy for you is because they have all those vital micronutrients.

The greatest thing we can do for our health is to get as many of those micronutrients as we can since they are needed in varying amounts and kinds. It's best to eat as many fruits and veggies as possible. And when you acquire your nutrients from natural sources like this, it is extremely difficult to overdo it.

Additionally, be very skeptical of food packages that claim to be "one of your five a day." There's a good likelihood the food has been heavily processed and no longer contains many nutrients. It is most certainly far lower in fiber, at the very least.

As a result, you won't get the same advantages as you would have if you had eaten that vitamin directly. When feasible, use common sense and consume as many whole, authentic fruits and veggies as you can!

The Perils of Overindulging in Fruits and Vegetables

Having said that, taking an excessive amount of fruits and vegetables might be harmful to you. Or, to put it a little more precisely, eating too much fruit may be harmful rather easily.

This is due to the fruit's strong acidity and high sugar content. It is particularly harmful to your teeth because of both of these factors. A lot of individuals who adopt diets that emphasize smoothie consumption can eventually have severe dental issues!

Avoiding consuming excessive amounts of fruit juice or smoothies is one way to address this. Vegetable smoothies, on the other hand, are usually much lower in sugar. The fact that fruits and vegetables still contain calories should also be taken into account. This is particularly true for items like avocados, which are now quite popular. Avocados may make you fat even though they are good for increasing testosterone (because of their beneficial saturated fat content) and helpful for those seeking to cut down on carbohydrates.

The misconception that "fruits and vegetables are healthy and therefore cannot make you fat" must be avoided.

In actuality, they still include calories, and to prevent unintended weight gain, you must continue to monitor and control those calories.

CHAPTER 8

FORMING A VEGETABLE AND FRUIT-RICH DIET

You should thus strive to increase your intake of fruits and vegetables. As we've previously seen, many individual foods have very noteworthy health benefits, and there are also many specific vitamins and minerals that you should aim to include in your diet. However, what is the process for carrying out that plan? How do you go from not being able to eat your recommended five a day to being able to consume a wide variety of healthful components with ease?

Amazing strength of vegetables and fruits.

Because that's the second important realization you should have: you shouldn't be searching for each item separately in a reductive manner. You will discover that if you do this, you wind up paying a significant sum of money and get little return on investment.

Numerous fruits and vegetables that you may especially look for to reap advantages for your appearance, energy levels, immunity, inflammation, and other conditions are described in this book. As a result, you may be persuaded to believe that you may choose whatever perks you want! However, this strategy is incorrect.

You really cannot search out each superfood separately when there are THAT many different kinds of superfoods, each offering some kind of incredible advantage. This is particularly true considering that a lot of them are inedible for a limited period, many don't combine well, and many aren't on non your neighborhood grocery stores. What then do you do in its place?

The Plan: Diversification is the goal

It is better to just try to get as much diversity as you can in your diet rather than searching for certain types of fruits and vegetables. By doing this, you will include the widest variety of foods in your diet and, as a result, get the greatest variety of health advantages. Even if you found the world's healthiest superfood vegetable, you wouldn't gain anything from eating it since you would just be consuming enormous quantities of the same components.

Although we don't think of foods like apples as superfoods, they are just as spectacular as those more exotic concepts since they contain huge levels of epicatechin (a compound that creates serotonin, increases nitric oxide synthesis, enhances testosterone, and is an antioxidant).

Furthermore, you'll obtain a considerably wider variety of nutrients if you consume three different fruits and veggies.

Research indicates that a diverse diet is particularly beneficial for our microbiome, which consists of the beneficial bacteria that reside in our stomachs. Your gut health will be healthier the more variety of foods you consume, which will lead to weight reduction, more energy, improved mood, and other benefits.

Lastly, you may lessen the amount of thinking this diet boost requires by limiting your goal to just "eat lots of fruits and vegetables." This will increase your likelihood of sticking to your new commitment.

Guidelines for Expanding the Variety of Fruits and Vegetables

So how may the diversity be increased? Here are a few quick strategies to help you do that without making your next shopping trip too stressful:

• Cook a ton of Italian food, stews, and hot pots. It's extremely simple to simply put a lot of fruits and veggies into a pot with some mince when making something like bolognese.

• Try chopping carrots (so you don't have to peel them) and using frozen veggies like sweet corn, peas, and mushrooms to make this even simpler.

• Prepare a ton of salads! To create a simple cold lunch, just grab some salad leaves, add some sweet potatoes, cucumber slices, and a squeeze of lemon. You can serve this with almost anything you make. Selecting baby leaf spinach will provide you with iron and folate. Then just switch up which leaf you use each time.

• Refrain! When doing this, prepare a lot of food in bulk and freeze it in several Tupperware portions. Then, when it's time to eat, all you have to do is thaw each one.

Amazing strength of vegetables and fruits.

• Blend beverages! Making these is very simple; simply add a lot of fruits and/or veggies and mix. They also provide a plethora of incredible advantages. Smoothies are a staple diet for some of the happiest and most active individuals I know!

• Purchase fruits and vegetables. Fruits are often sold at counters in cafés and shops alike. Rather than purchasing a chocolate-flavored treat, just choose the most exotic-looking fruit you can locate!

CHAPTER NINE

WHAT IS THE CASE FOR MULTIVITAMIN SUPPLEMENTS?

If the vitamins, minerals, and other vital micronutrients found in fruits and vegetables are the primary sources of health benefits, then you may be wondering, "What about multivitamins?"

A supplement with a variety of nutrients balanced in one dose is called a multivitamin supplement. Usually, one that has a mix of vitamins C, D, A, and B complex will be visible. Similarly, for "healthy bones and hormone balance," multimineral supplements may include Iron, Magnesium, Potassium, Calcium, and Zinc.

Are these goods comparable to the "real deal" in quality?

Indeed and no.

You can, on the one hand, absorb supplements and get benefits from them. There are several solid reasons to think differently, despite what some individuals may tell you. To start with, did you know that several items on the market may completely replace your diet? These include products like Soylent, which is said to provide every nutrient the body needs in an ideal proportion.

Is this a smart move? In no way! However, the important thing to remember at this point is that those who utilize this substance live, and they're really in quite good health! We can thus say with certainty that multivitamins can also be absorbed in light of this.

There's a catch, however. The first of these traps is that the quality of a multivitamin depends only on the creator. As we saw, for instance, with lutein and other fat-soluble vitamins. To be absorbed into the circulation, they need a supply of fat. If you get them from whole food sources, the fat source will likely be disclosed. They may not if you get them from a vitamin supplement.

Amazing strength of vegetables and fruits.

Numerous other vitamins and minerals also interact similarly, facilitating the easier absorption of the other. Similarly, various vitamins and minerals should preferably not be mixed into a single product since they absorb at varying rates.

Then there are all the other healthy ingredients that fruits and vegetables have, such as fiber, amino acids, and other things. In addition, it should be noted that every fruit and vegetable has ingredients that we may not even be aware of or do not completely comprehend.

The remarkable (and beyond eye health) advantages of lutein are still relatively new to us. Therefore, it is always better to consume actual fruit and vegetables.

Having said that, if the decision is between taking a supplement and consuming no nutrients at all, the supplement is superior. As a "backup," supplements may be a very practical and simple approach to ensure that you are getting enough of the necessary nutrients in your diet.

CHAPTER TEN

YOUR BLUEPRINT FOR BETTER HEALTH

We have now concluded this tutorial. You should now have a much better understanding of the specific fruits and vegetables you need to eat, which ones may provide the most health advantages, and how diversity is more important than anything else.

In the same manner, you want to know how to include those fruits and veggies into your diet as well as how to steer clear of any potential problems.

Having said that here's your guide to eating more fruits and veggies for a major improvement in your health and happiness:

• Have a smoothie first thing in the morning, but limit yourself to one fruit smoothie.

• Don't limit your diet to just five to seven fruits and veggies. Acquire as many as you can to ensure a diverse blend.

• As a "backup," use a supplement. This is particularly helpful when looking for uncommon and hidden nutrients.

• However, be careful to follow the directions and do independent research. To help with absorption, you may want to consider timing and include a source of fat.

• Employ techniques to make including more fruits and vegetables in your diet as simple as possible.

Amazing strength of vegetables and fruits.

• Steer clear of processed meals and "empty calories"; in their place, eat carrot sticks and salads instead of chocolate bars and chips.

• Keep up this routine for a full 30 days. You ought to discover that your health has improved and that you have more vigor and drive.

• Make additional improvements to your lifestyle with this newfound vitality!